ESSENTIALS OF PHYSIOTHERAPY CLINICAL PRACTICE

A Guide for Physiotherapist

By

DR. AIMAN NIAZ PT

DPT, MS-Orthopedic Manual PT (RIU),
Certified Rehabilitation Pilates
(Australian Physiotherapy & Pilates Institute),
Clinical Head, Department of Physiotherapy,
The Physio Networks SBM Trust.

PREFACE

Being a clinician and in a busy work routine, one of the hardest things to do is to regularly practice things at which you are uncomfortable or less skilled. I have been working as a Consultant, supervising internships and trainings of physiotherapy professionals as well as students for 3 years and working as a content writer for 7 years. I had participated in many short courses over this period. And while supervising physiotherapy training programs I got to know the weaknesses in physiotherapist's clinical practice that needs to be improved and this emphasizes me to write this book to guide clinicians and students in their clinical practice. As most of all, not knowing how to practice all of your knowledge in a clinical setting. With the information in this book I hope to remove some of the uncertainty for physiotherapists.

This clear, readable text delivers "need to know" content, along with the essential basis to follow in physiotherapy clinical practice that physiotherapists need to succeed in their future careers. It is a powerful tool, and a pocket guide to help you in following clinical practice:

- Take you through role of physiotherapy profession and its responsibilities

- Presents key clinical concepts for assessment documentation

- Provides a logical, clinically reasoned approach to write physiotherapy prescription

- Evidence base approach to write case study

- Guidelines to follow in oral case presentation

- Emphasizes a physiotherapy diagnosis based on patient's/ client's level of functioning

Aiman Niaz

CONTENT

Preface	iii
Acknowledgements	iv
CHAPTER ONE Physiotherapy Profession and Responsibilities	1
CHAPTER TWO Physiotherapy Assessment Documentation	10
CHAPTER THREE Physiotherapy Case Study Writing	17
CHAPTER FOUR Physiotherapy Oral Case Presentation	23
CHAPTER FIVE Physiotherapy Prescription Writing	31
CHAPTER SIX Physiotherapy Diagnosis	35
CHAPTER SEVEN Physiotherapy Areas of Practice: Key Points **A- Musculoskeletal Physiotherapy** **B- Neurological Physiotherapy** **C- Cardiopulmonary Physiotherapy** **D- Electrotherapy**	40 41 69 86 105
References	111

Chapter One

PHYSIOTHERAPY PROFESSION & RESPONSIBILITIES

A Guide to Physiotherapy Profession & Responsibilities

"Physiotherapy" and "physical therapy" and the terms "physiotherapy" and "physical therapy" are synonyms.

Physiotherapist (PT) is a clinician / health care professional who diagnoses and treats people of all ages, from neonates to the geriatric population, who have medical problems or other health problems that limit their ability to move and perform functional activities in life.

Physical therapy can only be provided by qualified physiotherapists (PT) or Physical Therapist Assistants (PTA) who work under the supervision of a physiotherapist.

Responsibilities of Physiotherapy Department

The physical therapy department is responsible for:

— Proper ordering, maintenance, and storage of all physical therapy equipment and supplies.

- All record keeping associated with patient care.
- Inspection of all equipment for safety and cleanliness.
- Performance of daily start-up and shut-down of automated physical therapy equipment.
- Training of clinic staff in physical therapy procedures.
- Review and update of physical therapy Policy and Procedures Manual annually.
- Quality control, quality assurance, and risk management as they relate to physical therapy functions.

Responsibilities of Physiotherapist

- Every patient should be assessed thoroughly on the first day of assessment.
- The initial assessment done and treatment given should be documented on the same day.
- Plan of care for each patient should be designed taking into consideration patients' current physical levels, prior levels, and their goals from physiotherapy.
- Goals, short term or long term should be set for each patient. These goals should be documented at the time of initial assessment.

- Treatment session details for each patient should be documented on a daily basis.
- Progress note for each patient should be documented after every 6 days
- Each patient should be reassessed/re-examined after 15 days or 10 sessions whichever comes first.
- For the patients assessed by trainee PT/ junior physical therapist, each initial assessment and one treatment session each week should be supervised by the respective senior therapist.
- Therapists should not be allowed to use mobile-phones/ electronic gadgets during session.
- Therapist should be responsible to coordinate with HR to manage patient's time.
- The PT should perform a follow up evaluation every two weeks or after 15 treatment sessions whichever comes first.
- The patient should be referred back to the appropriate medical provider if no improvement is noted within two weeks of starting physical therapy.
- Physical therapists show respect and sensitivity to people and communities, taking into account

their spiritual, emotional, social and physical needs.

A physiotherapist (only) shall conduct an evaluation, documenting the following

- History, chief complaint or other pertinent information
- Subjective data
- Objective and evaluative data
- Assessment
- Plan of treatment
- Frequency and duration of treatment and follow-up plan

Physiotherapy Assistant

PT assistant should:

— Perform physiotherapy plan of care after the patient has been evaluated/examined by the senior physical therapist.
— Perform his/her duties under the direction and supervision of the physical therapist.
— Perform administrative functions within the department including patient appointments and patient records

Physiotherapy Policies and Procedures

Documentation

The physiotherapist (PT) documents all sorts of information regarding patient / client management, including initial evaluation / examination and assessment, diagnosis, prognosis, treatment, response to interventions, changes in status due to interventions, review and disposal / discontinuation of intervention.

The physiotherapist makes sure that the documentation is used properly, ensuring that it is safely stored at all times, in accordance with the legal privacy and confidentiality requirements of personal health information and only released when appropriate with the patient's/client's permission.

Initial Examination, Assessment, Diagnosis

The physical therapist performs an initial examination / evaluation and assessment to establish a diagnosis and prognosis / plan prior to intervention / treatment. The examination must be documented, dated, and appropriately authenticated by the physical therapist who performed it may result in recommendations for additional services to meet the needs of the patient/client.

Plan of Care

Based on the assessment of the patient's physical, cognitive, emotional and social condition, a written treatment plan is developed that identifies the needs of patients for physiotherapy. The plan includes at least:

- Patient's personal goals for rehabilitation.
- The objectives and goals of physiotherapy related to daily life activities, functional activity and working level.
- Measures and deadlines for achieving physiotherapy objectives.

Intervention/Treatment

Interventions/treatments should be provided by physical therapist

The physical therapist provides the physical therapy intervention/treatment consistent with the results of the examination, evaluation, diagnosis, prognosis and plan of care/intervention/treatment.

When interventions/treatments are provided by trainee physical therapist or by physiotherapy assistant they must be provided under the ongoing direction and supervision of the senior physical therapist.

Re-examination

The physical therapist re-examines the patient / client, as appropriate, every 15 days to assess the progress or change of patient / client status, and modifies the plan accordingly or discontinues physical therapy services.

Discharge / Discontinuation

The physiotherapist discharges the patient / client from the physical therapy services when the expected outcomes for the patient / client has been reached.

The physiotherapist discontinues the treatment when the patient / client cannot progress toward goals or when the physical therapist determines that the patient / client no longer benefits from physiotherapy.

Patient / client collaboration

In the patient / client management process, the physiotherapist and the patient maintain a continuous process of collaborative decision-making that exists throughout the delivery of services.

Referral

Where the examination, diagnostic process or any change in status reveals findings outside the scope of knowledge, experience or expertise of the physical therapist, the physiotherapist should refer the patient/client to the appropriate practitioner.

Personal/professional development

The physiotherapist is responsible for individual professional development and should maintain a high level of professional skill by continued participation in various learning experiences.

Quality assurance

The physiotherapy service must have a written plan for continuous improvement of quality of care and performance of services.

Research

The physiotherapist should advance the science of physical therapy by conducting and supporting research activities or by assisting those engaged in research.

Functions and Services

Patient satisfaction Surveys

Patient satisfaction forms are administered to more than 90% of all the patients coming to the physiotherapy dept. These data are collected on a daily basis. These physiotherapy-specific forms are then scored and analyzed on a monthly basis to assess the levels of patients' satisfaction.

Patients Feedback forms

These forms are to be filled by each patient on last treatment session or on monthly basis. These forms too are scored, and the data analyzed monthly.

Chapter Two

PHYSIOTHERAPY ASSESSMENT DOCUMENTATION

A Guide to Assessment Documentation

(examination, evaluation, diagnosis, prognosis and plan of care including interventions)

Documentation is a very important process in physiotherapy practice.

It's a skill that needs to be perfected as the correct assessment leads towards correct diagnosis.

First introduce yourself

Before getting data from your client, you should always introduce yourself and make him or her comfortable talking to you. If possible, the area should be free of distractions. This could probably make the person feel more comfortable talking to you.

SOAP Method for documentation

SOAP notes are a highly structured format to document the assessment and progress of a patient during treatment and is one of the many possible formats that could be used by a health professional to enter the patient's /clients medical data and to communicate information to other care providers to provide evidence of contact with patients and to inform the clinical reasoning process.

SOAP is an acronym for:

1. **Subjective** - What the patient says about the problem / intervention.

2. **Objective** - The physiotherapist's objective observations and treatment interventions

3. **Assessment** - Analysis of the various components of the assessment.

4. **Plan** - How the treatment will be developed to the reach the goals or objectives.

Subjective Examination

Subject: Patient Name, Age, Occupation

Chief Complaint/Ailment/Injury

Date of Injury/ Date of Surgery

History of Present Illness (HPI)
In the history of present illness, or HPI, you will be asking questions that are related to the specific problem of your client. This may include asking:
What made you come here?
What did you feel? Please describe to me

(Location/Intensity/Duration) or describe other symptoms you feel?
What were you doing or What was your activity when your symptoms occurred?
What makes your symptoms better or What makes it worse?
What did you do about your symptoms? (Consultations, Medications and treatments provided including relevant lab works and results if available)
What other problems do you have?
Pain and dysfunction score (NPRS)

If your patient's /client's symptoms had been present in the past then ask why he/she decided to have a consultation today.

Use of the mnemonics OLD CARTS, that stands for Onset, Location, Duration, Character, Aggravating factors, Relieving factors, Timing and Severity.

But as you become skilled in clinical questioning then questions that your supposed to ask will come in naturally.

Your Clinical Eye
Sometimes, you will know what your patient's /client's problem is before the actual evaluation and examination as the patient / client enters the evaluation room. This is your clinical eye working.

Example: Your patient / client is walking with exaggerated right hip and knee bending, lifting the foot to clear it off the ground during walking. You might expect that he has weakness/ paralysis of his muscles in front of the leg (ankle dorsiflexors). Since you know that could be the case with your patient / client, you can now prepare your questions in your mind.

Past Medical/ Surgical History (PMHx)
Ask about past medical conditions and the treatments they are having. Ask about previous surgery/surgeries that they had for any health problem.

Family Medical History
Some conditions are inherited. Sometimes, health problems, such as heart disease, osteoporosis and diabetes run in their family, putting them at risk for the condition, as well.

OBJECTIVE EXAMINATION

Observation
Posture, Gait, Edema, Muscle Wasting, Deformity, Pressure Sores, Wounds, External Appliances

Palpation
Warmth, Tenderness, Tone, Swelling

Tests and Measurements
During the initial evaluation, you will establish a baseline data by performing physiotherapy tests and measurements, which will become your basis for your physiotherapy treatment plan.

Essential test and measurements in your physiotherapy documentation may include:
Vitals: Blood pressure, pulse rate and temperature
Joint ROM (range of motion)
Manual muscle tests (MMT)
Other related measurements specific to your patient's / client's problem.

Special Tests
To determine the actual structure affected you may also need to perform special tests such as orthopedic special tests in musculoskeletal examination. For example, the Anterior drawer test, which can be used to test for anterior cruciate

ligament injury or the McMurray test for meniscus injuries.

Laboratory Investigations
(Such as CBC, ESR etc.)
Radiological Considerations
(Such as X-Ray, MRI, CT-Scan etc.)

Assessment

Assessment is a thought process that may not include formal documentation. It may include documentation of the evaluation of the data collected in the examination and identification of problems relevant to patient / client management.

Physiotherapy Diagnosis
It indicates level of impairment such as activity limitation and participation restriction determined by the physiotherapist.

Prognosis
Provides documentation of the expected level of improvement that can be achieved through the intervention and the time taken to reach that level.

Plan of care
It includes goals, planned interventions, proposed frequency and duration, and discharge plans.

Client / patient goal setting
Setting goals of physical therapy should involve the patient/client. Goals should be realistic and achievable according to the condition and problems of the person. By making your client actively participate in setting goals, they will feel more comfortable and more motivated to achieve those goals, resulting in better results.

Progress note or daily note
It includes documentation of the progressive implementation of the plan of care recognized by the physiotherapist, including changes in the patient / client status, and variations and progressions of specific interventions used. You can also include specific plans for the next visit or visits.

Re-examination Documentation
It includes data from new or repeated examination and is provided to evaluate progress and to modify intervention.

Discharge / Discontinuation Documentation
It is required following conclusion of the current sessions and summarize progression toward goals in the physical therapy intervention and discharge plans.

Chapter Three

PHYSIOTHERAPY CASE STUDY WRITING

A Guide to Case Study Writing

— Title page

— Abstract

— Introduction

— Case Presentation

— Management and Outcome

— Discussion

— References

Template

Title:
Running Header:
Authors:
Name, academic degrees and affiliation
Name, address and telephone number of corresponding author/authors
Statement that patient consent was obtained
Key words: (limit of five)
Abstract: (maximum of 150 words)

Introduction
Case Presentation
Management and Outcome
Discussion
References
Tables, figures or images

Title:

It should be expressive and brief as titles attract readers (Average between 8 to 9 words in length)

(Example- A case study: 'Mobilization with movement technique in cervicogenic headache')

Abstract:

— It includes a summary of the purpose, case presentation, management and outcomes.

— It has two styles, narrative or structured

— Narrative abstract- A narrative abstract consists of a summary of the whole paper like a story which flows logically. There are no headings in this abstract style.

— Structured abstract- A structured abstract uses subheadings. This style is becoming more popular for scientific and clinical studies as it standardizes the abstract and confirm that certain information is included.

Introduction:

— Provide background of the case and describe any similar cases which are reported previously.

— If there is anything challenging or interesting while diagnosing or managing the case that you are describing then it's worth mentioning in the introduction.

— Introduction has to be not more than a few paragraphs long, and its objective is to make the reader understand clearly that why it is useful for them to read this case.

Case Presentation:

— Introductory sentence: e.g. This 30-year-old female office worker presented for the treatment of low back pain.

— Describe the important nature of the complaint, including location, intensity, duration and associated symptoms: e.g. she is having asymmetrical right low back and right posterior thigh pain. Sometimes it radiates towards the right leg and foot. She describes the pain as having an intensity of up to 5/10. When the pain is particularly bad, she feels difficulty in walking.

— Further progress of history including details of time and circumstances of onset, and the evolution of the complaint: e.g. This problem began to develop 2 years ago when she slipped and fell down on the floor. Her back pain increased in frequency in the last year, now occurring four to five days per week.

— Describe aggravating and relieving factors. Also describe responses to other treatment: e.g. The pain seems likely to be worse at the end of the work day. The pain aggravated by bending and relieved by reclining. NSAIDS provides some relieve. She didn't go for any other treatment.

— Include other health history, if relevant

— Include family history, if relevant.

— Summarize the results of examination, which might include general observation and postural analysis, structural alignment, palpation, myotome tests, orthopedic exam, spinal AROM, lumbar repeated movements, neurological exam, reflex assessment, SLR measures, and spring testing. e.g. The postural exam revealed a decreased lumbar lordosis. Spinal flexion AROM was found to be within normal limits and was measured with a single inclinometer. Repeated flexion in standing and in supine caused the patient's symptoms to worsen in the right posterior thigh, while repeated lumbar extension in standing for 10 repetitions resulted in movement of the symptoms from the posterior thigh to the right low back indicating a centralization of symptoms. Further centralization of symptoms to the lumbar spine done by repeated extension in lying following 20 repetitions. Palpation revealed tenderness in the lumbar paravertebral bilaterally.

— The patient was diagnosed with mechanical low back pain. Physiotherapy diagnosis was functional limitation.

Management and Outcome:

— Describe the provided treatment as specifically as possible, including the nature of the treatment, and the frequency and duration of care: e.g. The patient undertook a course of treatment consisting of lumbar spinal manipulation three times per week for two weeks. Manipulation was accompanied by trigger point therapy to the paraspinal muscles and McKenzie exercises. Furthermore, advice was provided regarding maintenance of proper posture at work. The patient was also instructed in the use of a lumbar cushion.

— State objective measures of the patient's progress if possible, e.g. the intensity of her LBP declined throughout the course of treatment.

— Describe the resolution of care: e.g. Based on the patient's progress report during the first two weeks of care, she received an additional two treatments in each of the subsequent two weeks. During the last week of care, she experienced no back pain and reported feeling generally more energetic than before. Following a total of four weeks of care (10 treatments) she was discharged.

Discussion:

Summarize the case and any lessons learned: e.g. This case shows a classical presentation of mechanical LBP which resolved quickly with a course of spinal manipulation, supportive soft-tissue therapy and postural advice.

References: (using Vancouver style) e.g.

(Tables, figures or images)

Chapter Four

PHYSIOTHERAPY ORAL CASE PRESENTATION

A Guide to Oral Case Presentations

Oral Case presentation is an important skill for the physical therapy student to learn.

Once you have collected the data, you should be able to document it in a written format and pass it on clearly to other health care professionals. To do this successfully, you need to understand the patient's illnesses, psychosocial contributions and physical diagnostic findings. You then need to compress them into a concise and organized recitation of the most essential facts. The listener needs to receive all relevant information without the irrelevant details and must be able to construct his own differential diagnosis as the story unfolds. Consider an advocate who is trying to persuade an informed and interested judge about the merits of his argument without distorting any of the facts.

Basic principles

An oral physiotherapy case presentation is not a simple recitation of your notes (write-up). It is a concise and edited presentation of the most important information.

Length – this will vary-

— A full presentation in attending rounds should be under 5 minutes.

— A full presentation in a case discussion session in front of other healthcare providers under 15 minutes -10 for the presentation and 5 for questions.

Basic structure for oral physiotherapy case presentations

— **Chief complaint (CC)**

— **History of present illness (HPI)**

— **Other active problems**

— **Past medical/surgical history**

— **Brief social history (current situation and major issues only)**

— **Physical examination (pertinent findings only)**

— **One-line summary (Assessment and plan)**

Organization and Content of Case Presentation

Chief Complaint (CC) – your presentation should involve the listener and give them a feel for the patient as a person.

Structure: "Mr./Mrs./Ms. ___ is a ___year-old male/female who presents with a chief complaint of _____, or who visit to the clinic for follow up of_____)".

To guide your listener, identifying information should include the patient's relevant active complaints, which usually should not more than four. You will list these problems here only for diagnosis and will elaborate them later in history of present illness.

Example: Mr. Ali is a 40-year-old man who was electively admitted for evaluation of exertional dyspnea. His active problems include rheumatoid arthritis. He was in his normal state of health until...

Avoid presentation of distracting information, such as an overly detailed discussion of the patient's medical/physical problems in your introductory remarks.

History of Present Illness (HPI)

Introductory sentence:

Mr./Mrs./Ms.____ was in his/her usual state of ____ (e.g., poor health / excellent health) until ____ (e.g., five days prior to visit) when he/she developed the ___ (acute/gradual) onset of _____.

- The introductory sentence may include details of past medical/physical history if the patient's illness directly relates to an ongoing chronic disease.
- Don't mention that an event occurred on Monday, rather refer to the time relative to the day of admission, e.g. 3 days prior to admission.
- Content of HPI- specifically characterize the major presenting symptoms including patient clinical features, any prior complications.
  The following is a useful mnemonic to make sure all those bases are covered:

- **C** character, circumstances
- **L** location – deep or superficial, well or poorly localized
- **E** exacerbating factors
- **A** alleviating factors

- **R** radiation of pain
- **A** associated symptoms
- **S** severity on a 1-10 scale
- **T** temporal features - timing (intermittent / constant), changes over time (progressive, stable or improving), duration, frequency.

Other Medical Problems

- Include here details of those problems that are active and you feel are relevant to the present illness. These are usually the same problems you mentioned in "chief complaint". For example, adhesive capsulitis is relevant to a patient came with stroke. Each condition should be considered separately, recounting the details in a chronological order. In other words, first explain the patient's h/o adhesive capsulitis, telling the story from the beginning to the present and then discuss stroke.

- Key words and phrases summarize a chronic disease in progress if they are related to the current problem, as explained above. In general, keywords emphasize the date of diagnosis, treatment, current symptoms, complications, and any recent objective tests.

— In the case presentation you avoid presentation of irrelevant diagnoses. For example, malaria in 2015 are probably not relevant during presentation of the rheumatoid arthritis.

Past Medical/Surgical History

— Provide a list of all prescribed medications and associated allergies. Report as much detail about drugs/medications as the patient can give you.

— Report any previous surgery/surgeries in chronological order. For example, patient had right TKR (total knee replacement) 5 years ago.

— Provide details of metal implants used in any surgical procedure. For example, metal implants used in fracture repair.

— Summarize substance use not already mentioned in HPI. However, if it has been mentioned in the HPI, do not repeat it.

Social History

Please do not try to reduce patients just to habits and marital status as we are more than these facts. Summarize your social history in a brief paragraph (two to three sentences) commenting on current life situation, including work, and support systems and any ongoing social issues. It is often the social history that explains why the patient has fallen ill now, e.g. patient having low back pain may be associated to his occupation. For example, if he is working in a factory.

Physical Examination

— General description – describe in such a colorful way that it allows the listener to visualize the patient. For example, the patient was sitting on a wheelchair, leaning forward and gasping for breath due to pain.

— Vital signs should always be mentioned.

— Special Test and Investigations

— Mention only the relevant positive findings and relevant negative findings.

> **Summary and Assessment (brief)**
>
> It should present in this pattern: "...the patient's major presenting problem is _____ (best positive statement you can make; say "low back pain" and avoid statements like "rule-out disc bulge"). The differential diagnosis includes _____, _____, and _____. The diagnosis of _____ appears to be the most likely of these because _____.

Chapter Five

PHYSIOTHERAPY PRESCRIPTION WRITING

A Guide to Prescription Writing

Prescription writing in physiotherapy clinical practice needs a lot of skill and experience.

Here are some specific rules and pattern to consider for writing physical prescriptions.

You will prescribe therapy much like as you would prescribe a medication. You must know the patient, the problem you are addressing, the concurrent problems that may affect your prescription and what the goal is

Use the therapy as if it were your bag of tricks based on your skills to achieve the treatment goals. The physical therapy prescription should a careful goal-oriented approach rather than a mindless cookbook recipe approach. (Don't just copy and paste)

Be careful to consider every word in your prescriptions in order to avoid over-writing as well.

The correct and balanced prescription writing is more like an art that takes years of experience with the therapists and patient populations

It is helpful to think about the following questions

- Which structures are weak that need to be strengthened?
- which structures are tight that need to be stretched or elongated?
- Which movements are poorly coordinated or have biomechanical flaws that need to be retrained and corrected?
- What types of manual therapy techniques would be effective?
- What therapeutic modalities are safe and useful for my patient/client?
- What other impairments exist?
- Which activities or positions should be encouraged to promote recovery?
- Which activities or positions needs to be avoided due to their detrimental effects?
- What training and educational resources would be useful for my patient?

Rx

Name with identifying factors
(e.g. the patient's name, date of birth, medical record numbers etc., along with the date the prescription was written.)

Diagnosis
— Begin with your primary diagnosis, then secondary diagnoses if relevant.

— Identify contributing factors to the diagnosis (e.g., tight hamstrings in the setting of mechanical low back pain).

— Body part and side to be treated

— Relevant past medical and surgical history.

Problem list (Complaint of....)

Assessment finding
(e.g. Special tests, labs, radiograph findings)

Precautions/recommendations
(e.g. avoid stair climbing, cross leg sitting and use commode)

Frequency of visits
(such as 2 to 3x/week)

Duration of treatment
(Such as 3 to 4 weeks; or 8 to 12 total visits)

Therapeutic modalities
(Such as heat packs/cold packs, electrical stimulation)

Manual therapy
(Such as manipulation, trigger point release, massage)

Therapeutic exercise
(Such as AROM/ AAROM/ PROM, stretching, strengthening, balance/proprioceptive training or conditioning exercise)

Specialized treatments
(Such as kinesiology taping, Pilates)

Patient education
(Such as written home exercise programs)

Goals
(Such as decrease pain and swelling, restore ROM and flexibility then strength, or safely return to functional activities, e.g. work)

Reevaluation
(Such as 3 to 4 weeks by referring physician)

Chapter Six

PHYSIOTHERAPY DIAGNOSIS

A Guide to Physiotherapy Diagnosis

Diagnosis

The information the physiotherapist receives about the patient is information provided by the patient or the data provided by a referring physician which could be a medical diagnosis or a symptom diagnosis.

Medical diagnosis

The medical diagnosis may be a disease-diagnosis, such as rheumatoid arthritis, cerebrovascular accident, multiple sclerosis or parkinson's disease (classified according to the International Classification of Diseases and Related Health Problems). The diagnosis may also be a symptom-diagnosis, especially in cases where the GP or medical specialist cannot specify the disorder or disease. For example, dysfunction of the neck and back, headache, dizziness, or referred pain in the arm are symptom-diagnoses.

Process of physiotherapy diagnosis

The Physiotherapist gathers information from the clinical history and by physical examination in order to gain insight into the health condition and perceived health problem. Or it could be based on the medical diagnosis, the referral diagnosis, and the referral data.

A physical therapist unlike a physician, addresses needs of each patient differently. Hence, there is a need to change from the previous followed traditional medical approach for physical therapy diagnosis to the movement dysfunction approach.

In physiotherapy practice, patient presents with complaints related to functions, which are usually forgotten in documentation of pathological model that emphasizes on the diagnosis of diseases. While ICF Bio-psychosocial model used by physical therapists comprehends the physical body, mental state, and the social characteristics in continuity with the WHO definition of Health.

The main objective of the physiotherapy diagnostic process is to obtain an impression of the pathway from disease to the nature and intensity of the health problem/ condition, and the extent to which these may be acted upon. It is expected that this pathway progresses from pathology or disorder, to impairments (dysfunctions), to disabilities (restriction in elementary and/or complex activities), to restriction in (social) participation and to quality of life.

THE ICF MODEL

(ICF -The International Classification of Functioning, Disability and Health)

The ICF is a biopsychosocial model of disability, conceptualizes a person's level of functioning as a dynamic interaction between her or his health conditions, environmental factors, and personal factors and supported by The World Confederation of Physical Therapy (WCPT).

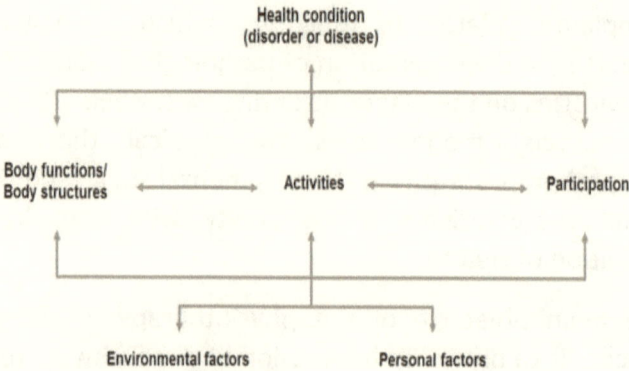

Body Functions and Structures

— **Body functions**: The physiological functions (including psychological functions) of body systems

— **Body structures**: Anatomical structure of the body such as limbs, organs and their components

- **Impairments:** Problems in functioning at the level of the body and structure such as significant deviation or loss

Activities and Participation

- Activity: The execution of a task or functioning at the level of the individual
- Activity limitations: Difficulties which an individual may have in performing activities
- Participation: the participation or Involvement in a life situation
- Participation restrictions: Problems an individual may experience in involvement in life situations (functioning of a person as a member of society)

Environmental Factors

The environmental factors such as physical, social and attitudinal environment in which people live and conduct their lives. These are either facilitators or barriers to the person's functioning.

For example, products and technology, natural environment & human-made changes to environment, support and relationships, attitudes, values and beliefs, services, system and policies

Personal Factors

— Personal Factors should also be considered in the model but are not classified within the actual ICF framework

— For example, Personal factors: gender, education, personality, coping styles, life habits, social background

THE DIAGNOSTIC PROCES

HEALTH CONDITION (disorder/disease) (e.g. Spinal Cord Injury)			
Function impairment (e.g. Problems of muscle power and structure of spinal cord)		**Activities limitation** (e.g. Difficulty moving and walking)	**Participation restriction** (e.g. Restricted participation in employment and in using public transport)
Environmental factors (e.g. Public transport, barriers in building design)		**Personal factors** (e.g. Male, 40 yrs.)	

Chapter Seven

PHYSIOTHERAPY AREAS OF PRACTICE: KEY POINTS

A Guide to Physiotherapy Clinical Practice Areas

- A- Neurological Physiotherapy
- B- Cardiopulmonary Physiotherapy
- C- Musculoskeletal Physiotherapy

Physiotherapy is a wide-ranging profession with many different areas to practice including musculoskeletal, neurological, cardiopulmonary, pediatric, women health, geriatric and sports physiotherapy. Here is a guide of specific topics which a physiotherapist needs to learn before starting practice in three major physiotherapy areas (musculoskeletal, neurological and cardiopulmonary physiotherapy).

First of all, learn basics of SOAP (Subjective, Objective, Assessment, Plan) notes and know the basics about the specific area of physiotherapy. For example, if you started practice in musculoskeletal then know the basic, revise and practice specific practical skills about musculoskeletal physiotherapy (e.g. special tests, goniometry).

A- Musculoskeletal Physiotherapy

- Learn about basic anatomy and surface marking of the spinal column, peripheral joints, major muscle groups and ligaments
- Basic knowledge of bone and soft tissue healing
- Knowledge of pathology (osteoarthritis, rheumatoid arthritis, adhesive capsulitis etc.)
- Musculoskeletal assessment (Normal ROM of peripheral joints, capsular patterns, nerve tension tests, dermatomes, myotomes, reflexes and appropriate special tests)
- Fracture classifications, mechanisms of injury, surgical procedures and complications of fracture.
- Types of joint replacement
- Red and yellow flags
- Outcome measures for pain and peripheral joints (e.g. oxford muscle scale, goniometry)
- Electrotherapy (heat and cold therapy, ultrasound, TENS etc.)
- Types of gait patterns and use of walking aids

ROM of Different Movements of Major Joints	
Shoulder joint	— Forward flexion : 180 degrees — Extension : 45-60 degrees Abd : 180 degrees — External Rot : 90 degrees — Internal Rot : 70-90 degrees
Elbow joint	— Elbow flexion: 0 to 145 degrees — Forearm supination: 0 to 85 degrees — Forearm pronation: 0 to 80 degrees
Wrist complex	— Extension (dorsiflexion): 0 to 70 degrees — Palmar flexion: 0 to 80 degrees — Radial deviation: 0 to 20 degrees — ulnar deviation: 0 to 45 degrees
Hip joint	— Flexion: 0 to 125 degrees — Extension: 0 to 30 degrees — Adduction: 0 to 25 degrees — Abduction: 0 to 45 degrees — External rotation: 0 to 60 degrees — Internal rotation: 0 to 40 degrees

Knee joint	— Flexion: 0 to 140 degrees. — Extension: 0 degrees
Ankle joint	— Dorsiflexion: 0 to 20 degrees — Plantar flexion: 0 to 45 degrees

Manual Muscle Test Grades	
Grade 5 (Normal; 100%)	— The patient can complete the whole range of motion against gravity with maximum resistance applied by the therapist at end-of-range.
Grade 4 (Good; 75%)	— The subject can complete the whole ROM against gravity with moderate resistance applied by PT at end-range.
Grade 3+ (Fair+)	— The patient can complete the motion against gravity with minimal resistance applied by therapist at end-range.

Grade 3 (Fair;50%)	— The patient can only complete the ROM against gravity. When external force is applied by the PT, the patient gives way.
Grade 2 (Poor;25%)	— Patient can perform the movement only when pull of gravity is eliminated. No resistance is applied.
Grade 1 (Trace)	— Patient is not able to move the joint, not even when the gravity is eliminated. However, there is slight muscle contraction feels on palpation.
Grade 0 (Zero; No trace)	— No contraction is noticed, even with therapist's palpation.

Musculoskeletal Examination of the Shoulder	
OBJECTIVES	— Surface anatomy
	— Glenohumeral (GH) joint ROM
	— Cervical spine ROM
	— Acromioclavicular (AC) joint

	— Sternoclavicular (SC) joint — Subacromial bursa, rotator cuff, and biceps tendons — Special Test
Shoulder Examination from Front	
Observe and Inspect	Deltoid and pectoralis muscles, deltopectoral groove
ROM	Cervical spine
Palpate	SC joints, AC joints, biceps tendon, anterior subacromial region/bursa, lateral subdeltoid region/bursa
Resisted and Special Test	— Resisted shoulder abduction: supraspinatus test ("empty cans") — Resisted shoulder ER: rotator cuff integrity — Neer's impingement sign: passive shoulder flexion — Resisted supination of the forearm: Yerguson test — Hawkins impingement sign: passive shoulder flexion, adduction, and forced LR
Shoulder Examination from Behind	
Observe and Inspect	Supraspinatus, infraspinatus, and deltoid muscles

ROM	Active arm elevation and scapular motion
Shoulder Examination in Seated or Supine Position	
Observe and Inspect	— Shoulder flexion — Shoulder abduction — Shoulder external rotation and internal rotation
Special Test	Apprehension test
COMMON SHOULDER PROBLEMS	
Impingement	— Causes: overhead activities, throwing. — Repetitive forward flexion and abduction of the arm result in compression of the subacromial bursa, supraspinatus tendon and biceps tendon, and causes subacromial bursitis, supraspinatus tendonitis, and biceps tendonitis. **Subacromial Bursitis** — Pain occurs during arm elevation — Irritation and inflammation — Pain referred down the upper arm (deltoid region) to the mid-humerus

	Rotator Cuff Tears/Supraspinatus Tendonitis/Rotator Cuff Tendinitis — Sports related repetitive activity and overuse injury may result in irritation, inflammation, and tears of the rotator cuff. — Pain occurs during active or resisted abduction . — Pain radiates down the upper arm (deltoid region) to the mid-humerus. — Most common acute or chronic tear: supraspinatus and — Less common: infraspinatus **Biceps Tendonitis** — Pain during forward flexion and forearm supination. — Pain usually located anteriorly in the region of the bicipital groove.
Adhesive Capsulitis (Frozen Shoulder)	— Adhesive capsulitis is a condition refers to the globally decreased shoulder range of motion. — It is progressive and could

	be painful (early stage) or painless (late). — Passive ROM is diminished in all planes. — It could occur in association with stroke, diabetes mellitus, shoulder bursitis or tendonitis. — Plain x-rays of the shoulder are normal.
Glenohumeral Arthritis	— GH Arthritis presents with dull, diffuse, aching discomfort and swelling. — Restricted AROM: painful — Passive range of motion: painless — GH joint: crepitus on ROM — Plain x-rays show features of arthritis: joint space narrowing, osteophyte formation, sclerosis.
Cervical Spine Referred Pain	— The neck frequently refers pain to the shoulder presenting as "shoulder" pain.

	— Non-radicular cervical pain. — Radiates along the trapezius.
Instability	— Patients has prior history of trauma or recurrent episodes of subluxation/dislocation or generalized joint hypermobility. — Patients complains as arm slipping out of joint. — Most common anterior instability. — Apprehension with certain movements especially combined Abd and — ER).

Musculoskeletal Examination of the Knee	
OBJECTIVES	— Surface anatomy — Patellofemoral and tibiofemoral joints — Medial collateral, Anterior, posterior cruciate, and lateral collateral ligaments — Medial and lateral menisci — Prepatellar and anserine bursae — Special test

Knee Examination from front	
Observe	Check knee alignment
Knee Examination in Supine Lying Position	
Observe and inspect	Inspect quadriceps, prepatellar bursa, medial, superolateral, and suprapatellar regions.
Palpate	Palpate medial, lateral patellar facets, anserine bursa and joint line.
ROM	Perform Flexion and extension of knee
Special Test	— Perform patellar apprehension test (push/pull patella laterally) — Lachman test (to check ACL, LCL, MCL, PCL) — Ant/posterior drawer test) — McMurray maneuver (To Check menisci)
COMMON KNEE PROBLEMS	
Arthritis of the Knee	— Patient's clinical history, age, gender — Pain, stiffness, swelling, crepitus, — Osteoarthritis: cool effusions

	— Rheumatoid arthritis, and psoriatic arthritis: cool to warm effusions — Septic arthritis: warm effusions
Patellofemoral Pain Syndrome	— Patellofemoral pain is characterized by diffuse, dull, aching, ant knee. — Pain that increases with activities such as ascending or descending stairs, prolonged sitting, kneeling and squatting. — More common in women than men. — Tenderness on patellar facets palpation. — Weakness of the quadriceps muscles
Prepatellar Bursitis	— Swelling of the prepatellar bursa result from chronic, frictional irritation to the bursa due to excessive kneeling, bacterial infection, crystalline inflammation or direct trauma causing inflammatory bursitis, septic

	bursitis, gouty bursitis, hemorrhagic bursitis respectively.
Collateral Ligament Tear (Sprain)	— The collateral ligaments are the primary stabilizers of the knee against varus and valgus stresses and could occur alone or in association with anterior/ post cruciate ligaments or med/lateral meniscal injury. — MCL injury may occur if sudden valgus force is applied to the lower extremity, driving the tibia laterally into abduction. — LCL injury may occur if sudden varus force is applied to the lower extremity, driving the tibia medially into adduction. It is less common than MCL injury.
Cruciate Ligament Tear (Sprain)	— The cruciate ligaments are the primary stabilizers of the knee against. — Post (PCL) and ant (ACL) stresses, preventing

	translation of the tibia on the femur.
	— ACL injury may result from a sudden twisting or hyperextension of the knee, causing the ligament to tear. It gives feeling of giving away and causes early hemorrhagic knee effusion. ACL injury is mostly associated with MCL and meniscal injury (called "unhappy triad")
	— PCL injury (less common than ACL injury) may result from a sudden force applied to the anterior tibia, driving it posteriorly with the knee in flexion.
Meniscal Tears	— The medial and lateral menisci are fibrocartilages, acting as a shock-absorber and internal-stabilizers of knee which may be torn as the result of acute traumatic injury.
	— Meniscal tears usually result from a significant twisting injury or chronic

	degeneration, causing acute pain, swelling and stiffness and Mechanical symptoms of popping, clicking or locking of the knee.

Musculoskeletal Examination of the Neck	
OBJECTIVES	— Surface anatomy — Cervical ROM — Myofascial trigger points and tender points (fibromyalgia) — Cervical myelopathy — Suspected cervical nerve root irritation
Neck Examination	
Observe and Inspect	— Observe posture, alignment, movement, and inspect skin.
Palpation	— Palpate occiput and spinous processes, myofascial trigger points or tender points (fibromyalgia), scapular borders.

Range of Motion	— Cervical spine flex, ext, lateral bending and rotation.
Special Test	— Screening of suspected shoulder pathology. — Reflexes: Biceps (CS), brachioradialis (C6), triceps (C7) — Resisted test to check muscle strength. — Dermatome, myotome. — Spurling test: apply gentle pressure to occiput during combined rot and ext to the affected side. Considered positive if reproduces radicular pain.
COMMON NECK PROBLEMS	
Acute Neck Pain	— Acute uncomplicated neck pain is a common, usually self-limited disorder. — Patient experiences pain from sharp to aching in quality, but no radiation to the upper limb

	— Pain may occur prolonged periods of cervical flex /ext / rotation, or wrong sleep positioning, or after athletic injury, or minor trauma.
Whiplash Injury	— Whiplash is a mechanism of injury of the C spine occurs most frequently secondary to athletic injury or motor vehicle accidents. — Acceleration and deceleration forces causes injury to intervertebral disks and paraspinal soft tissues causing discomfort cervical region with referral to shoulders. — If causes spinal fracture, or dislocation then patient should be referred for orthopedic assessment.
Cervical Spondylosis	— Commonly occurs in older individuals related to the degenerative changes of the vertebral bodies, loss of the integrity of the intervertebral disk,

	secondary osteoarthritic changes are referred to as cervical spondylosis. — It causes reduced cervical ROM and local neck pain which sometimes referred to the shoulders or scapulae. Stiffness and crepitus on motion, positional pain, and sleep difficulty may also be present.
Cervical Radiculopathy	— Cervical radiculopathy usually results from nerve root irritation due to disk herniation or facet joint hypertrophy. — Cervical pain combined with neurogenic pain which referred to the upper extremity.
Other Less Common Neck Problems	— Cervical Myelopathy — Spondylarthritis — Chronic Neck Pain — Malignancy — Referred Visceral Disease — Infection

Musculoskeletal Examination of the Low Back	
OBJECTIVES	— Observation of gait, posture. — Inspection, palpation, and ROM of the lumbosacral spine. — Examination and evaluation of the hip, sacroiliitis and suspected nerve root irritation. — Consideration of systemic or visceral disease.
Observe and Inspect	— Observe posture, gait, alignment, movement, curvature and skin.
Palpation	— Palpate spinous processes and skin tenderness, trochanteric bursa, gluteus medius insertion
Range of Motion	— Lumbosacral: flex, extension, side bending and rot — Hip: flex, extension, internal and ext rotation
Special Test	— Reflexes: Patellar reflexes (L4), Achilles reflexes (Sl) — SLR Test (Straight Leg Raising)

	— Muscle Strength and Sensation testing — FABER test (hip flex, abduction, and external rot) — Iliac compression test (on superior anterior iliac spines)
COMMON LOW BACK PROBLEMS	
Acute Low Back Pain	— Acute uncomplicated low back pain usually occurs due to lifting or bending activities and can be felt in the lumbar spine, LS junction, post thighs and buttock without radiating below the knees. — It is a common, self-limited, but frequently recurrent problem.
Lumbosacral Radiculopathy	— LBP combined with neurogenic lower extremity pain (sciatica) due to lumbosacral nerve root irritation. — Pain radiates from the buttock to the posterolateral thigh to the ankle/ foot.

	— May be sudden or gradual in onset.
Lumbar Spondylosis	— Commonly occurs in older individuals related to the degenerative changes of the vertebral bodies, loss of the integrity of the intervertebral disk, secondary osteoarthritic changes are referred to as lumbar spondylosis. — LS movements may be painful and limited, especially lateral flex and extension. — Pain is mechanical in nature which aggravated with activity and relieved by rest.
Lumbar Spinal Stenosis	— Spinal stenosis is disc disease, relatively common in old individuals and generally occurs due to loss of disk height resulting in narrowing of the spinal canal. — It causes pain with tingling or numbness in one or both legs and relieved by sitting or spinal flexion.

Other low pain problems	— Chronic Pain Syndrome — Osteoporotic Compression Fractures — Spinal Fractures — Malignancy — Visceral Disease Infection

Common Treatment Techniques	
Maitland Geoff Maitland is an Australian physiotherapist who transformed the teaching of vertebral manipulations.	— Grade I: Small amplitude movement without resistance — Grade II: Large amplitude movement with small amounts of resistance — Grade III: large amplitude into range. — Grade IV: Small amplitude in range, right at the end of the joint range — Grade V: This is a manipulation rather than a mobilization Lower grades are aimed at pain and the higher grades are aimed at range of movement.

McKenzie Robin McKenzie is a physiotherapist from New Zealand who formed a spinal treatment from it that is widely used by physiotherapists today.	The idea is to centralize the pain by exercises in a posterior disk hernia. It is suggested that, an extension biased exercises express pressure over the posterior aspect of the disk, providing pain relief by forcing the gelatinous nucleus pulposus back into a central position.
Mulligan Brian Mulligan is a New Zealand physiotherapist.	The concept behind this technique is providing a sustained parallel or perpendicular glide to a joint to the end of pain free range to increase the overall range of movement. Two types of movement considered by the concept. — Sustained natural apophyseal glides (SNAG) – a vertebral mobilization. — Mobilization with movement (MWM) – a passive accessory movement with active (or

	passive) physiologic movement of the joint.
Muscle Energy Techniques (MET)	— Reciprocal inhibition is simply the fact that contraction of an agonist will exert an inhibitory effect upon the contraction of its antagonist. E.g. Elbow – during biceps contraction (which acts as agonist), the triceps (which is antagonist) relaxes and allow additional force to be expressed over it (i.e. a stretch). — Postisometric relaxation works by the principle that maximal contraction is followed by maximal relaxation.
Myofascial therapy Dr Travell 1st used the terminologies	The technique is simply a soft tissue manipulation that releases the myofascial that allows normal healing to occur.

which we use today – trigger point and myofascial therapy.	
Pilates Introduced by Joseph Pilates as a method of rehabilitation.	Pilates is an excellent aide to the other physiotherapy techniques for all types of patients as it not only encourages better core stability, it also give control to the patient, over their condition, and that is probably the most effective treatment you can give. It also encompassed breathing techniques to deliver high quantities of oxygen to the tissues.
Exercise Therapy	— Passive movement — Active Assisted exercise — Active movement — Resisted exercise — Stretching exercises — Isometric and strengthening exercises

Exercise Therapy Equipments	— Static cycle — Treadmill — Parallel bar — Tilt table — Quadriceps table — Shoulder wheel Abduction ladder — Hand exerciser — Medicine ball — Wheelchair — Crutches

\multicolumn{2}{c}{**GAIT**}
\multicolumn{2}{c}{Human gait refers to locomotion attained through the movement of human limbs.}
Pathological gait	— Antalgic gait — Festinent gait — Circumductory gait — Scissoring gait — Ataxic gait — High stepping gait

Gait training	**Types of weight bearing**
	— **Non-weight bearing**
	  Do not weight through involved leg.
	— **Partial weight bearing**
	  Maximum 50% of the body weight applied to the involved leg.
	— **Weight bearing**
	  Allow as much weight as tolerated through involved leg.

	Use of Crutches
Standing up with crutches	— Slide hips forward to the edge of the bed, chair or toilet seat. — Keep injured/healing leg straight and healthy leg beneath — Place both crutches in the hand of injured/ healing leg bearing no weight. — While standing, reach with free hand for the other crutch and then place both crutches under armpits with hands firmly holding the handgrips
Walking with crutches	— While walking forward both crutches approximately one foot ahead while balancing weight on healthy leg. — Step forward with injured/healing leg first. — Then step forward healthy leg, bringing it through the crutches and after the injured/ healing leg — Remember to keep weight on your hands

Climbing stairs with both crutches	While Climbing stairs Remember this statement " Climb up stairs with the good leg first and down stairs with the bad first"

B- Neurological Physiotherapy

— Neurological conditions you will come across including pathology, signs and symptoms, medical and physiotherapy management. (e.g., Parkinson's disease, multiple sclerosis, stroke, Guillain–Barre' syndrome, etc.)

— Neurological assessment (i.e. ROM, tone, sensation, muscle power, posture, balance etc.)

— Outcome measures (i.e. Berg balance scale, motor assessment scale).

— Types of physiotherapy treatments which are used by physiotherapist for specific types of neurological conditions. (e.g. balance re-education, exercise prescription).

Disease Specific Considerations for Examination

Parkinson's Disease	
Examination	
Pathophysiology:	Progressive loss of dopamine in the basal ganglia.
Basal ganglia's role	Initiates, stops, monitors and maintains movement. Functions as a "braking system" to inhibit undesired movement and permit desired ones.
4 Cardinal Signs	1. Tremor 2. Rigidity (Cog Wheeling) 3. Bradykinesia 4. Postural Instability
Coordination Testing	— Finger Tapping — Mass grasp — Pronation/Supination — Toe tapping
Things not affected	Strength, sensation, cranial nerves (though many have loss of smell as an early symptom)
Balance Considerations	Loss of automatic postural control

Parkinsonian Gait	1. Shuffling (Short step length bilaterally, flexed forward at hips, often lack arm swing unilaterally). 2. Festinating gait (Unable to control forward movement of trunk which leads to falling. 3. Freezing
Outcome Measures	
Considerations for testing	— Timing of medications. — Practice effect - gait speed, 2 min walk. — Note quality of movement, not just time.
Gait Measures	2/6 min walk test 10 m walk test
Balance Measures	Functional Gait Assessment
Functional Strength	5x sit to stand
Subjective Outcome Measures	— ABC scale — Parkinson's Disease

	Questionnaire - 8 or 39 — Freezing of Gait Questionnaire
Treatment	
Patients are classified into Hoehn & Yahr stages- treatments vary depending on progression of disease	— Hoehn & Yahr 1 & 2: Limited postural instability, early diagnosis. Primarily ambulatory without device. — H&Y Stage 3: Begin to have postural instability by demonstrating lack of recovery on pull test. — H&Y Stages 4-5: Severe disability (Stage 4 can still ambulate, stage 5 is wheelchair bound).
Goals	— Delay progression through education and early mobility training. — Educate on exercise and initiate program. — Perform thorough examination of appropriate outcome measures for baseline and to detect areas needed

	for training.
	— Treat specific impairments (Freezing, festination, shuffling, etc.) as they become more prevalent.
	— Within session learning improves with use of cues.
	— Continue high intensity training, progressive aerobic exercise as able.
	— Start early and provide a lot of repetition to reach automaticity.
	— Parkinson's Disease Specific Home Exercise Programs.
	— Caregiver education.
	— Equipment as needed.
4 S's to follow	1. Stop 2. Standing tall 3. Sway 4. Step big

Multiple Sclerosis	
Examination	
Pathophysiology	Demyelination occurs in the central nervous system in the brain and/or spinal cord. Signs and symptoms will depend on the areas of demyelination.
Common Signs	— Sensory impairment with complaints of numbness or paresthesia in a cortical or dermatomal pattern. — Motor impairment in cortical or myotomal pattern. — Spasticity — Vision and oculomotor deficits including deficits in acuity, ocular alignment, and oculomotor. — Coordination and ataxia. — Dizziness — Fatigue - primary and secondary. — Bowel and bladder impairment (spasticity).

	— Heat sensitivity
	— Balance deficits >> falls
Classification of Disease	1. Relapsing Remitting: Individuals have relapses of symptoms and then recover. 2. Relapsing progressive: Have instances of increased symptoms with partial but not complete recovery. 3. Secondary Progressive: Initially have relapsing remitting but as the patient continues to progress in the disease course, have steady decline in function without periods of recovery. 4. Primary Progressive: Steady decline in function without periods of recovery from onset of disease.

Examination Considerations	— UMN signs, localization in cortex, brainstem, cerebellum, or spinal cord. — Cranial nerve evaluation, especially oculomotor. — Coordination testing: Ataxic, dysmetric movements if cerebellum is involved - (rapid alternating movements, finger to nose, heel to shin). — Tone assessment: Modified Ashworth Scale - expect hypertonicity. — Reflex assessment: Expect hyperreflexia, presence of abnormal reflexes - babinski and clonus. — Sensory Testing — Manual Muscle Testing — Cognition testing: Alertness and orientation. — Fatigue assessment: Modified Fatigue Impact

	Scale. — Complete vestibular exam. — Balance assessment: Likely to have poor sensory input as well as inability to produce good motor output. — Gait assessment: Impairments that will lead to gait deficits. — Common deficits seen: foot drop, steppage gait, circumduction, trendelenburg due to weak glute medius, Ataxia, wide BOS.
Outcomes Measures	
Considerations	Fatigue and timing of tests Environment factors- heat, time of day.
Gait Measures	— 6 min walk test — 2 min walk test — Timed 25-foot walk — Timed Up and Go with cognitive and manual components

Balance Measures	— Berg Balance Scale — Functional Gait Assessment
Fine Motor/Coordination	— Functional Strength — 5x sit to stand
Subjective Measures	— 12-item MS walking scale — Modified Fatigue Impact Scale — Fatigue Scale for Motor and Cognitive Functions — MS Impact Scale — MS Quality of Life
Treatment	
Goals of treatment	1. Relapsing Remitting — PT begins after steroids are initiated. — Rehab focused on impairments and functional limitations that occur with relapse. — Education on relapse prevention and recognition.

	— Provide necessary compensatory and supportive equipment.
	— Fatigue Management
	— Aerobic Exercise
	— Strength Training
	— Balance Training and Fall Risk Management
	
	2. Secondary and Primary Progressive
	    — Compensatory mechanisms
	    — Equipment Needs
	    — Caregiver training
	
	3. Other considerations
	    — Spasticity management
	    — Fatigue Management
	    — Cognitive Considerations
	    — Vestibular and Dizziness complaints
	    — Timing of treatment to allow for maximum

	functioning during day
Evidence Based Treatment	**Aerobic Exercise** — Consider role that fatigue may play in aerobic exercise. — Moderate intensity is best. — Manage environment to prevent overheating, encourage fluids to prevent overheating. — May be best done with walking, biking, or any aerobic medium patient feels comfortable. — Can help with overall management of disease. **Balance Treatment** — Static and dynamic training — Very important to train to prevent falls. — Fatigue may increase imbalance.

	Strengthening — Important to include strength training as part of program. — Include full body strength training. — Yoga and Pilates are good options. **Fatigue Management** — Energy conservation techniques. — Maximize gait efficiency and assistive device use to prevent extra energy expenditure with gait. — Regular exercise can decrease fatigue. **Vestibular Treatment** — Can improve postural control and balance. — Progressive exercises that incorporate head movement, eye movement, and balance on various surfaces.

STROKE	
Examination	
Pathophysiology	— Vascular event leading to damage of brain tissue supplied by that vessel (MCA, ACA, PCA).
Signs and Symptoms	— Vary significantly depending on vessel affected. — Most common: MCA, ACA, PCA. — Other common: lacunar, cerebellar, and vertebrobasilar.
Common Impairments to Examine	**Motor** — Loss in cortical distribution unilaterally >> hemiplegia. — UE often more affected than LE. — LE muscles often affected: dorsiflexors, quadriceps, hamstrings, and gluteus maximus. **Sensory** — Loss in cortical distribution in unilateral.

	— May be complete sensory loss or partial. — Test light touch, proprioception, sharp / dull. **Cranial Nerves** — Oculomotor impairment — Palate and uvula deviation — Tongue deviation — Facial droop with forehead/eyebrow movement preserved **Reflexes** — Hypertonicity unilaterally — Unilateral abnormal reflexes **Cognition** — Memory impairments — Emotional lability **Postural assessment** — Sitting and standing — Ability to sense upright — Even weight distribution left to right — Signs of pusher syndrome

	Speech deficits — Slurred speech — Aphasia **Balance evaluation** — Static and dynamic balance assessment is important. — Deficits with co-contraction of muscles, torque, and sequencing. **Gait Evaluation** — Circumduction — Steppage
Outcome Measures	
Considerations	Keep assistive devices consistent.
Gait Measures	— 6 min walk test — 2 min walk test — 10 m walk test — Timed Up and Go
Stroke Specific Impairment Scales	— Postural Assessment Scale for Stroke (PASS) — Stroke Rehabilitation Assessment of Movement (STREAM)
Balance	— Berg Balance Scale

Measures	— Functional Reach — Dynamic Gait Index — Functional Gait Assessment
Treatment	

Goals of Treatment (for cortical MCA/ACA)	— Early intervention
	    o Start rehab within first 24-48 hours
	    o Remember to check hypertension
	— Push neuroplasticity.
	— Aerobic activity to prevent future strokes.
	— Early gait and functional training.

Gait Training	— Weight shift — Perceived upright posture — High Intensity Training — Treadmill Training

C- Cardiopulmonary Physiotherapy

- Thoracic anatomy and surface marking.
- Knowledge of respiratory problems such as COPD asthma, pneumonia, pneumothorax, bronchitis and bronchiectasis.
- X-ray interpretation.
- Common types of surgery and surgical incision.
- Complications of surgery.
- Normal values for SpO_2 (blood oxygen levels), arterial blood gas, heart rate, respiratory rate and blood pressure.
- Types of mechanical ventilation.
- Basic knowledge of tracheostomy care.
- Treatment options e.g. ACBTs, spirometry, suctioning, positioning, postural drainage, bed mobility, manual techniques and oxygen therapy and cardiac rehabilitation.

Chronic Obstructive Pulmonary Disease

COPD is a general term that refers to a number of chronic pulmonary conditions characterized by narrowing and obstruction of airways, increased retention of pulmonary secretions and airflow limitation is progressive and not fully reversible.

Examination	
General Clinical Problems	— Dyspnea on exertion — Prolonged and labored expiration — Chronic accumulation of pulmonary secretions — Decreased endurance and exercise capacity — Associated postural defects
Classification of Disease	— Chronic bronchitis — Emphysema — Asthma — Other diseases such as cystic fibrosis and bronchiectasis usually lead to chronic obstructive dysfunction
Goals	— Relief of dyspnea — Removal of secretions — Improve exercise tolerance

Treatment Methods	
Relief of Dyspnea	— Relaxed Positions: The 1st step is positioning. It is an effective technique to reduce the symptoms of breathlessness. — Breathing Retraining Exercises: Breathing exercises relieve dyspnea and improve gas exchange. The techniques most commonly taught are pursed lips and diaphragmatic breathing or a combination of both. • Diaphragmatic Breathing Diaphragmatic breathing exercise improves the force of the diaphragm as an inspiratory muscle. It improves ventilation of small airways and bases of the lungs. • Pursed lips breathing (PLB): Pursed lips breathing exercise prevents collapse of airways during expiration by maintaining positive airways pressure during expiration.

	— Breathing Control Techniques: Breathing control techniques encourage deep breathing and control dyspnea. e.g. 1 step to breathe in and 2 steps to breathe out, or 1 for each.
Biofeedback and respiratory muscle training	— Biofeedback teaches self-control and as a result, it builds strength and endurance in the respiratory muscles. —Incentive spirometry: The goal is to encourage patient to take deep breathing which leads to reduction of breathlessness. —The oximetry can use as a biofeedback guide to teach patient to increase their oxygen saturation during performance of pursed lips breathing.
Secretion Clearance	— Huffing and Coughing: Patients are trained and encouraged to 'cough' or

| | 'huff' and clear secretions effectively. It opens glottis minimize collapse of small airways. |
| | — Chest physiotherapy: Postural drainage, percussion, vibration |

Guidelines for exercise prescription for patients with COPD	
Aerobic Exercises	— Mode: Walking, cycling, swimming etc. — Frequency: 3 to 5 times per week. — Intensity: Another approach is to exercise at maximum limits tolerated by symptoms or 50% of peak VO_2 (minimum). — Duration: 20 to 30 min (minimum) of continuous exercise.
Flexibility Exercise:	Stretching of major muscles as a part of the warm up and cool down before and after aerobic training.
Strengthening Exercise	Strength training in specific muscle groups as weakness of muscles is common in COPD.

	Restrictive Lung Diseases
	Are group of diseases, all characterized by decrease in pulmonary ventilation, deep breathing and lung expansion.
Aetiology	— **Pulmonary causes** Tumor, pneumonia, atelectasis, heart disease or fibrotic lung disease. — **Extrapulmonary causes** Postural deviations (i.e. kyphosis, scoliosis), pleural effusion, or chest wall stiffness due to pulmonary or cardiac surgery. — **Respiratory muscle weakness** Neuromuscular disease i.e. parkinsonism, muscular dystrophy.
Pathomechanism	Any of the above-mentioned causes affect mainly the lung expansion and lead to decreased the lung compliance and lung volume which increase the work of breathing of respiratory muscles

	especially the diaphragm.
Signs and Symptoms	Dyspnea, hypoxemia, tachypnea, cough postural deviations, muscle wasting and, weight loss.
Treatment	
Goals	—Relief dyspnea and pain —Correct postural defects —Increase chest expansion —Improve exercise tolerance
Exercises	—Respiratory exercises (i.e. deep breathing ex), AROM, stretching, positioning and gym exercise —Endurance exercises (walking, cycling, swimming and treadmill training — Modalities for pain relief (e.g. TENS, infrared or laser)

	Role of physiotherapy in cardiothoracic surgery
Goals	— Adequate ventilation. — Removal of excess secretions — Post-operative venous thrombosis prevention — Prevention of postural defects — To maintain shoulders and spine mobility
Pre-operative training	Explanation to the patient about the procedure and taught exercises to patients which he has to perfume after surgery — Removal of secretions — Breathing exercises — Huffing and coughing — Ankle pumping ex — Shoulder girdle and arm movements — Postural guidance
Post-operative treatment	**Day of operation** If the patient is not on a ventilator and cardiovascular system is stable then as soon as he is conscious enough to co-operate

breathing exercises should be started on the day of the operation.

1ˢᵗ and 2ⁿᵈ day after operation

Physiotherapy sessions four times a day

— Breathing exercises

— Ankle pumping

— Huffing and coughing

— Shoulder movements

Third day onwards

— As the patient starts sitting out of bed and as per surgeon's instructions, walking should be started around the ward.

— The exercises performed on 1ˢᵗ and 2ⁿᵈ day should be continued. Trunk exercises and postural correction should be added.

— 6 days from the time of operation walking upstairs can usually be started

Before discharge

Patient will probably be

	discharged after 10-14 days when exercise tolerance increases and thoracic expansion, posture and shoulder mobility should have returned to normal.

Complications Following Cardiothoracic Surgery

Factors that increase the postoperative complications	— General anesthesia — Intubation — Pain medication — Incisional pain — General weakness due to inactivity and bed rest
Complications	— Cardiac problems — Respiratory problems — Thrombosis — Wound infections — Pressure sores — Muscle wasting

Respiratory problems: Atelectasis, postoperative pneumonia, pulmonary embolism, hypoxia

Physiotherapy Goals	To regain the normal vital capacity and full use of the lungs
Methods	— Effective coughing

	— Breathing exercises
	— Removal of secretions

Deep venous thrombosis

DVT is a clot of blood that remains at the site of origin, if it detaches can travel to the right side of the heart and can enter the lung called a pulmonary embolism.

Physiotherapy	**Prevention:** Instruct the patient before operation about ankle pumping and deep breathing exercises at least for five minutes/ every hour and postoperative leg mobilization (ankle pumping). **If DVT developed** — In acute cases physiotherapy is contra-indicated. — In chronic cases • Control swelling and aid venous return by applying elastic bandage. • Deep breathing

	exercise. • Active exercise.
Pressure sores Prevention: Changing the patient posture frequently, check the integrity of the skin and areas of redness.	
Neurological damage Physiotherapy must be performed to treat any form of paralysis if occurs during cardiac surgery as the brain may be damaged by embolism or anoxia.	

Cardiac Rehabilitation	
Cardiac rehabilitation is a therapeutic process designed to facilitate maximal restoration of function and to achievable goals.	
Objectives	— Relief of cardiac symptoms
	— Improved exercise tolerance
	— Reverse pathophysiologic effects of heart disease
	— Improved psychosocial well being
	— Improvement in the blood levels of lipids
	— Reduced mortality
	— Reverse the atherosclerosis by establishing exercise training programs and education, counseling
Indications	— CABG (Coronary bypass)
	— Recent myocardial infarction
	— Valve surgery
	— Coronary angioplasty
	— Cardiac transplantation

Contraindications	— Uncontrolled arrhythmias — Severe residual angina — Uncompensated heart failure — Poorly controlled hypertension — Severe ischemia or arrhythmia during exercise testing
Phases of cardiac rehabilitation: 4 phases	
Phase I (Immediate inpatient phase)	— It is the acute in hospital phase — 7-14 days in duration — The goal is to start early physical therapy activities Exercises: — Active and passive ROM — Ankle pumping — Warm-up exercises — Stretching — Walk at slow pace and back, starting from 50 ft bid, then proceed to 75 ft bid, then few stair steps. — Reach up to 300 to 500 ft bid

Phase II:	— Phase II starts on an outpatient basis immediately after hospitalization — 8-12 weeks in duration — The goal of this phase is to increase exercise capacity and endurance — Conditioning exercises — Specific monitoring: HR, BP, ECG, sign and symptoms — Return to work
Phase III: **Outpatient** **(Home program)**	— Patients takes follow up from physiotherapist and do their exercises independently during phase — 6 months to one year in duration — The goal is to improve exercise fitness at high exercise intensity. Home Program — Daily walk — 26 to 8 hours sleep every night.

	— Wait at least one hour after meals before exercising.
Phase IV	— It is lifetime maintenance phase, in which physical fitness and reduction of other risk factors are emphasized.
Exercise prescription of cardiac patients	— Based on the results of the exercise stress test (prescribed in METs).
	— The Borg scale of Rate of Perceived Exertion (RPE).
	Prescription
	Mode
	— Aerobic exercise training includes walking, running, jogging, swimming and stationary bicycling.
	Frequency
	— Multiple short sessions/day for individuals with < 3-MET capacity.
	— 1-2 sessions/ day for individuals with a 3-5

	MET capacity.
	— 3-5 sessions /week for individuals with > 5-MET capacity.
	Duration
	— 30-60 minutes for each session, including 10 minutes warm-up and 10 minutes cool-up.
	Intensity
	— The intensity prescribed according to target heart rate.
	Exercise session consists of:
	— Warming-up:10 minutes
	— Aerobic exercise: 40 minutes
	— Cooling down: 10 minutes

Role of Physiotherapy in Intensive Care Unit	
Goals	— Assist in secretions removal
	— Improve ventilation of lungs
	— Maintain good posture and mobility of the patients
	— To decrease patient's hospital stay
Techniques	— Breathing exercises and incentive spirometer
	— Postural drainage, percussion and vibrations
	— Tracheal suctioning, coughing
	— Mobilization techniques

D- Electrotherapy

Low and Medium Frequency Modalities	**Low Frequency** Frequency of 1-1000 Hz **Medium Frequency** 1000-10.000 Hz — TENS (transcutaneous Electrical Nerve Stimulation) — Neuromuscular Electrical Stimulation — Galvanic Stimulation — Interferential Therapy (I.F.T) — Russian current — Faradic current Iontophoresis
High Frequency Modalities	**High frequency** Those current of 10,000 Hz or more. — Shortwave Diathermy (S.W.D) — Ultra Sound Therapy (U.S)

	— Microwave Diathermy (M.W.D)
Thermotherapy Moist and Dry Heat	**Benefits** — Alleviates pain by reducing endorphins when applied. — Increases white blood cells, stimulating an immune system response. — Reduces muscle spasms. — Increases blood volume, oxygenation, and nutrition.
Ultrasound Therapy	Therapeutic ultrasound has the frequency range of about 0.8 to 3.0 MHz. **Benefits** — Ultrasound other than just the potential heating effect, can produce many effects. — Increases local blood flow, tissue relaxation, and increases scar tissue breakdown. — Promotes bone fracture healing.

	Treatment Time
	— 3 to 5 minutes which depends on the size of the area being treated.
	Conditions Treated
	— Tendinitis , non-acute joint swelling, muscle spasm, and to break down the scar tissue.
	Contraindications
	— Local malignancy, metal implants, local acute infection, vascular abnormalities, and directly on the abdomen of pregnant women
Short wave Diathermy	Its frequency is 27,120,000 cycles/second and the wavelength is 11m.
	Indications
	— Inflammation of shoulder joint
	— Tennis Elbow
	— Osteoarthritis
	— Plantar fascitis
	— Degeneration of joints of neck (Cervical Spondylosis)

	— Ligament Sprains in knee joint — Low Back Ache **Treatment Time** — Initial Stage - 5-10 minutes — Moderate Stage - 10-20 minutes — Severe State - 20-30 minutes **Advantages** — Relaxation of the muscles — Relief of pain — Effective in bacterial infections
Interferential Therapy	IFT (Interferential Therapy) uses a mid frequency current for treatment. **Indications** — Pain — Muscles spasm — Muscles strain — Swelling **Contraindications** — Localized wounds

	— Recent cuts — Skin infection — Unhealed scar
Transcutaneous Electrical Nerve Stimulator	TENS unit is usually connected to the skin using 2 or more electrodes. — Sensory intensity: TENS is applied at high frequency (>50 Hz) with an intensity below motor contraction — Motor intensity: Low frequency (<10 Hz) with an intensity that produces motor contraction. **Conditions Treated** — Bursitis — Arthritis — Tendonitis — Headaches and migraines — It is also used for injuries and wound **Benefits** TENS unit sends electrical pulses through the skin. These pulses control pain signals in the body, causing temporary or permanent

	pain relief.
Cold pack	The effects of ice packs include pain relief, prevention of swelling and bruising, and decreased blood flow.
Wax bath	Paraffin Baths (122 – 130o Fahrenheit) **Benefits** Paraffin wax treatments are used to apply heat energy to the tissues. The petroleum-based waxy mixture is white and odorless and conforms well to wrists, hands, feet, ankles, knees, and elbows. **Conditions Treated** Paraffin is used for pain relief and softening the skin. Paraffin baths are used for arthritic joints or bursitis, except when joints are hot and swollen.

REFERENCES

Chetty, L. (2014) 'A Critical Review of Physiotherapy as a Clinical Service in Occupational Health Departments', *Workplace Health & Safety*, 62(9), pp. 389–394. doi: 10.3928/21650799-20140804-01.

https://www.apta.org/PTCareers/RoleofaPT/

Jump up ↑ SOAP note. (2019, May 15). In Wikipedia, The Free Encyclopedia. Accessed May 15, 2019

Zimny NJ. Diagnostic classification and orthopaedic physical therapy practice: What we can learn from medicine. J Orthop Sports Phys Ther. 2004;34:105–9. [PubMed] [Google Scholar]

Budgell B. Guidelines to the writing of case studies. The Journal of the Canadian Chiropractic Association. 2008 Dec;52(4):199.

Childs, J.D. (2004). Case reports: can we improve? Journal of Orthopedics and Sports Physical Therapy, 34, 44-46.

Guide to Physical Therapist Practice (Rev 2nd ed). (2003). Alexandria, Va: American Physical Therapy Association.

Ther Umsch. 2014 Jun;71(6):324-34. doi: 10.1024/0040-5930/a000520.

https://www.nyspmr.org/wp-content/uploads/2014/03/Dr.-James-Wyss_guide-to-PT-prescription-writing_Chapter-07_Basics-of-Musculoskeletal-Rehabilitation.pdf

World Health Organization. ICF Checklist Version 2.1a, Clinician Form. 2003. Available at: http://www.who.int/classifications/icf/training/icfchecklist.pdf

American Psychological Association Procedural Manual and Guide for the Standardized Application of the ICF: http://www.apa.org/monitor/jan06/changing.aspx

WHO Family of International Classifications http://www.who.int/classifications/en/

Stucki G, Reinhardt JD, Grimby G, Melvin J 2007. Developing 'human functioning and rehabilitation research' from the comprehensive perspective. J Rehabil Med 2007; 39: 665-671

Sykes C. Health classifications 1 - An introduction to the ICF. WCPT Keynotes. World Confederation for Physical Therapy. 2006.

Electro Therapy explained - Principle and Practice John Low & Ann Reed

Tidy's Physiotherapy-Ann Thomson, Alison Skinner & Joan Piercy

Rauch A, Cieza A, Stucki G. How to apply the International

Classification of Functioning, Disability and Health (ICF) for rehabilitation management in clinical practice. Eur J Phys Rehabil. 2008;44(3):329-42.

Hurst R 2003. The international disability rights movement and the ICF. Disability and Rehabilitation Vol 25, No, 1112, 572-576

Carter S K, Rizzo J A 2007 Use of outpatient physical therapy services by people with musculoskeletal conditions. Physical Therapy 87 (Mar 20 [Epub ahead of print]).

Clare H A, Adams R, Maher C G 2004 A systematic review of efficacy of McKenzie therapy for spinal pain. Australian Journal of Physiotherapy 50(4):209–216.

Klippel]H, Stone jH, Crofford Lj, White PH. Primer on the Rheumatic Diseases. 13th ed. New York, NY

Springer; 2008.

Lawry G, Kreder HJ, Hawker J, jerome D. Fam's Musculosheletal Examination and joint Injection Techniques.

2nd ed. Philadelphia, PA: Mosby/Elsevier; 2010.

Glover W, McGregor A, Sullivan C, Hague J 2005 Work-related musculo-skeletal disorders affecting members of the Chartered Society of Physiotherapy. Physiotherapy 91:138–147

Borton D C, Walker K, Pirpiris M et al 2001 Isolated

calf lengthening in cerebral palsy. Journal of Bone and Joint Surgery 83B:364–370. Bunker T 2002 Rotator cuff disease. Current Orthopaedics 16:223–233.

Shaieb M D, Kan D M, Spencer K et al 2002 A prospective randomized comparison of patella tendon versus semitendinosus and gracilis tendon autografts for anterior cruciate ligament reconstruction. American Jour-nal of Sports Medicine 30: 214–220.

Skinner J S P 2005 Exercise Testing and Exercise Prescription for Special Cases, 3rd edn. Lippincott, Williams and Wilkins, London.

Standring S 2005 Gray's Anatomy, 39th edn. The Anatomical Basis for Clinical Practice. Elsevier, Edinburgh.

Allingham C, McConnell J 2003 Conservative management of rotator cuff, capsulitis and frozen shoulder. In: Prosser R, Conolly W B (eds), Rehabilitation of the Hand and Upper Limb. Butterworth Heinemann, Edinburgh, p. 241–250.

Alvarez-Nemegyei J, Canoso J 2004 Evidence-based soft tissue rheuma-tology: III: trochanteric bursitis. Journal of Clinical Rheumatology 10 (3):123–124.

Partridge C 2002 Neurological Physiotherapy: Evidence Based Case Reports. John Wiley & sons London.

NICE (National Institute for Clinical Excellence) 2004 Beta interferon and Glatiramer acetate for the treatment of multiple sclerosis. Oaktree Press, London.

Nieuwboer A., de Weerdt W, Dom R et al 2000 Development of an activ-ity scale for individuals with advanced parkinson disease: reliability 'on-off' variability. Physical Therapy 80(11):1087–1096

Stokes M (ed) 2004 Physical Management in Neurological Physiother-apy, 2nd edn. Churchill Livingstone, London.

Weiner W J, Goetz C G 1994 Neurology for the Non-Neurologist, 3rd edn. Lippincott, Williams & Williams, Philadelphia.

Whitney S, Wrisley D, Furman J, 2003 Concurrent validity of the Berg Balance Scale and the Dynamic Gait Index in people with vestibular dys-function. Physiotherapy Research International 8(4):178–186.

Koninklijk Nederlands Genootschap voor Fysiotherapie 2005 Guidelines for physical therapy in patients with Parkinson's disease available from http://www.cebp.nl/?NODE=69 date accessed 14/9/07.

Lassmann H, Bruck W, Lucchinetti CF 2007 The immunopathology of multiple sclerosis: an overview. Brain Pathology 17(2):210–218. Lennon S 2003 Physiotherapy practice in stroke rehabilitation: a survey. Disability and Rehabilitation. 25(9):455–461.

National Collaborating Centre for Chronic Conditions 2004 Chronic obstructive pulmonary disease: management of chronic obstructive pul-monary disease in adults in primary and secondary care clinical guide-line 12. Thorax 59(suppl 1):S1-S232 Available: http://www.nice.org.uk/pdf/CG012_niceguideline.pdf 18 Feb 2007.

Cystic Fibrosis Trust 2002 Clinical guidelines for the physiotherapy management of cystic fibrosis. Cystic Fibrosis Trust, Bromley Available: http://www.cftrust.org.uk/aboutcf/publications/consensusdoc/ C_3400physiotherapy.pdf 18 Feb 2007.

Hough A 2001 Physiotherapy in Respiratory Care – an Evidence-based Approach to Respiratory and Cardiac Management, 3rd edn. Nelson Thornes, Surrey UK.

Chartered Society of Physiotherapy 2002 PA 53 Emergency respiratory on call working: guidance for physiotherapists. Chartered Society of Physiotherapy, London Available: http://www.csp.org.uk/uploads/documents/csp_physioprac_pa53.pdf 28 Feb 2007.

Hinds C J, Watson D 1996 Intensive Care – a Concise Textbook, 2nd edn. Saunders, London, p 183.

Hough A 2001 Physiotherapy in Respiratory Care – an Evidence-based Approach to Respiratory and Cardiac Management, 3rd edn. Nelson Thornes,

Surrey UK.

Stiller K, Phillips A 2003 Safety aspects of mobilising acutely ill inpati-ents. Physiotherapy Theory and Practice 19:239–257.

Orfanos P, Ellis E, Johnston C 1999 Effects of deep breathing and ambu-lation on pattern of ventilation in post-operative patients. Australian Journal of Physiotherapy 45:173–182.

Dhond, R.P., Yeh, C., Park, K., Kettner, N., Napadow, V., 2008. Acupuncture Modulates

Resting State Connectivity in Default and Sensorimotor Brain Networks. Pain 136,

407 – 418.

Hengeveld, E., Banks, K., 2005. Maitland's Peripheral Manipulation, Fifth ed. Butterworth-

Heinemann, Edinburgh.

Holey, E., Cook, E., 1997. Therapeutic Massage. WB Saunders, London.

Kisner, C., Colby, L.A., 2002. Therapeutic Exercise: Foundations and Techniques, Fourth

ed. F A Davis, Philadelphia.

Magee, D.J., 2008. Orthopedic Physical Assessment, Fifth ed. Saunders, Philadelphia.

Maitland, G., Hengeveld, E., Banks, K., English

Assessment Documentation

Case-1

S_____
_____
_____
_____

O_____
_____
_____
_____

A_____
_____
_____
_____

P_____
_____
_____
_____

Case-2

S_____

O_____

A_____

P_____

Case-3

S_____

O_____

A_____

P_____

Prescription Writing

Rx-1

Rx-2

Rx-3

Case Study_1

Case Study_2

Case Study_3

www.ingramcontent.com/pod-product-compliance
Lightning Source LLC
Chambersburg PA
CBHW030014190526
45157CB00016B/2702